My take on Reiki

By Jonathan Brandstater

For Lisa. Also, with thanks to Valerie, Nancy and others who have guided me on my healing journey. I am forever grateful.

List of topics

Introduction

Reiki is an alternative form of healing. It is an adjunct to Western Medicine. That is, Reiki can be used along with Western Medicine, specifically the use of medications, surgery and other treatments as appropriate but does not replace Western Medicine in any way. Broken bones still need to be set and wounds dressed. Reiki energy itself will help a patient feel better, without the side effects of medications. The term Reiki refers to Universal Life Force Energy. The method itself was developed by a Japanese monk named Mikao Usui in the early part of the twentieth century. One aspect of Reiki is the laying on of hands, using specific hand positions. In addition, there are other techniques, including distance or absent healing. One practitioner who has developed his own educational DVD uses his eyes to direct healing energy as well. Reiki itself is an art rather than a science. One brings his or her* own experience to the practice. There is also the traditional and non-traditional approach. The traditional approach includes most of the material Master Usui taught, as he taught it. The non-traditional approach allows for more leeway in terms of methods and techniques. I have often heard the expression: what we do is ninety nine percent intention and one percent technique. Keeping this expression in mind is very helpful.

Energy cannot be created or destroyed. It can only be transformed, that is, changed from one form to another. Matter itself is a dense form of energy. Reiki energy is everywhere and free. Anyone can access it, simply by breathing. Just about anyone can be a healer. A compassionate heart and a sincere desire to help people and be of service are important qualities. Also, just about anyone can learn Reiki or similar healing modalities.

Although I have practiced energy healing for over twenty years, I have been a Reiki master and practitioner since 2009. In addition, I have a minister's license. This allows me to discretely touch people, just as being a licensed physician allows physicians to touch people.

There are three levels of Reiki. For the first level, the student learns about the history of Reiki and also learns how to heal him or herself. This concept carries over into the second and third levels. One is only effective as a healer as he or she is healthy. Part of learning the history of Reiki includes mention of lineage. By lineage, I mean who taught Reiki to whom. We start with Master Usui and continue to the present teacher and the student. If I were to teach you Reiki, your Reiki lineage would include me as your teacher and the teacher who taught me, as well. There is also the consideration of whether the teacher taught the student in the traditional or nontraditional way. I myself am trained in the nontraditional approach.

At the second level, the student learns to heal others, both physically present and at a distance. At the third level, the student has the option of learning how to teach others.

The practice of Reiki includes the use of symbols. Some practitioners use the symbols taught by Master Usui while others use variations of the symbols. Symbols are useful in directing healing energy where it needs to go. There are no symbols for Level One Reiki. For Level two there is the power symbol, mental/emotional symbol and distance healing symbol. For Level three there is the Master symbol.

Attunements are part of teaching Reiki. Attunements are ceremonies. They might also be called initiations, where the student's energy channels are opened and maintained. The Reiki symbols are essentially passed from the teacher to the student. Perhaps the process needs a little explanation. In essence, the student's aura is opened and the symbols are drawn on his or her head and on the palms of his hands. He is encouraged to hold his hands to his heart as if to incorporate the symbols into his very being. One might consider attunements to be symbolic acts in and of themselves. As for auras, I will describe them in the next section.

*The use of the male pronoun is arbitrary. I do not mean to imply Reiki can only be practiced by men only. It is open to both genders. Writing "him or her" or "he or she" continuously is awkward.

Auras and chakras

The aura is an energy field. Every living thing has an aura. The energy field surrounds and pervades the entire body. Some mystics, psychics and clairvoyants can see auras. As a matter of fact, with practice, just about anyone can see them. Very likely, small children can see auras spontaneously. If a child says he sees colored lights around people, he is probably describing auras. Small children are open to experience and do not have the skepticism typical of some adults. Evidence for the existence of auras has been demonstrated through the use of what is called Kirlian photography. I have seen aura photographs of finger prints and leaves. The images galaxies. In addition, I have had aura photographs taken of myself, often with similar results.

Auras contain colors of the rainbow: red, orange, yellow, green, blue, indigo and purple. These are also colors of the visible spectrum. In addition, other colors may appear: gold, silver, white, brown, grey, black and color mixtures such as magenta and pink. According to some traditions, each color has a particular significance. Although one might associate red with anger, this is not always the case. It seems to depend on the hue and intensity. Red may also signify passion, will, courage, initiative and grounding (that is, being down to Earth and fully present). Orange signifies creativity. Yellow represents intellect. Green is associated with healing, as well as love and compassion. Blue signifies communication and indigo, intuition and clairvoyance. Purple represents connectedness to God, Goddess, Source or however one conceives a Higher Power. Brown denotes grounding. Grey may signify confusion and possibly disease. Black in the aura might suggest a blockage or something a person is holding on to. There is an application on smart phones and iPads called "iaura". You can take photos of yourself and/or other people and the app converts the images into "aura images" with interpretations. The suggested interpretation for black auras or black in a person's aura refers to holding onto to past hurts, anger and resentment. It also hints at the possibility of malice. In one book I read, the author speculates about black spots in the aura signifying "possible cancer." I consider this suggestion to be very risky. To speculate on a person's having cancer when none exists can have very unpleasant consequences. Magenta and pink signify unconditional love. Silver represents intuition, receptivity and the feminine principle. Gold denotes wisdom and the masculine principle. White, itself a combination of all colors, suggests spirituality and connectedness to Source, once again. In my case, when I think of unconditional love, I think of whole white light.

There are some commonalities between the practice of Yoga and the practice of Reiki. With yoga, there are references to auras and chakras. Each color is associated with a particular chakra. Chakra is Sanskrit for "wheel." The body is covered with chakras but there are seven major ones, each corresponding to a color, as well as to an endocrine gland and tone on the musical scale. Reiki includes seven hand positions, each corresponding to a chakra. As an aside, some healing modalities suggest there are between eight and ten chakras. At one workshop I attended, the facilitator advised us to visualize fourteen. Each additional chakra was the "finer," version of the ones below them. That is, the colors were lighter versions of the first seven chakras: from pink for the eighth chakra to bluish/white for the fourteenth. Speaking personally, I think seven major chakras are enough to consider.

The first chakra is called the root chakra and is located at the base of the spine, in the vicinity of the tail bone. This chakra is associated with survival and being grounded. The corresponding color is red and musical note is C. There is no gland associated per se associated with the root chakra but the anus is the site of elimination and "release" relates to survival and being grounded. The second chakra is called the sacral chakra, as well as "the bowl of creation." It is associated with creativity, sexuality and reproduction. The color is orange and note is D. The gonads and possibly also the adrenal glands are the corresponding endocrine glands. The third chakra is at the solar plexus. It is associated with the personal I, the ego, and intellect. The color is yellow and the note is E. The enteric (related to the intestines) gut might be the closest structure one can refer to in terms of endocrine glands, though the intestines themselves are organs rather than glands. The fourth chakra is located in the center of the chest, to the right of the heart. It is associated with connectedness to all living beings, as well as love and compassion. The color is green and note is F. The thymus surrounds the physical heart and might be considered the gland associated with the heart chakra. The fifth chakra is at the area of the throat. It is associated with the color blue. The note is G. The corresponding gland is the thyroid although one might also include the parathyroid glands. The sixth chakra is at the area of the forehead, corresponding to the third eye. It represents clairvoyance, intuition and dreaming. The color is indigo though some sources suggest it is purple. The pituitary gland corresponds to this chakra. The musical note is A. The seventh chakra is at the top of the head. It is also called the crown chakra and is associated with connectedness to God/Goddess/ Source/All that is. The color is either purple or white, depending on the source you consider. Speaking personally I associate the third eye chakra with indigo and the crown chakra with purple. The pineal gland corresponds to this chakra. The note is B.

Some practitioners work with animals, such as dogs, cats and horses. The chakra arrangements of these animals are similar to those of humans. Dogs, cats have front paws but no hands, of course. Horses have hooves. All these animals have chakras on their respective paws and hooves, as well as on and around their tails.

Exercises:

1. Gaze at the upper corner of a room. Allow your eyes to go out of focus. Do not stare,

squint or try to concentrate. As a matter of fact, do not "try" to do anything. Just observe. Very likely, you will notice a sort of shimmering cloud. This is energy. I've heard it described as "Chi". That is basically the same thing. You might want to do this exercise in a darkened room with a minimum of light or no light at all. Allow your eyes to get used to the darkness and then gaze up at a corner of the ceiling. Notice what you observe.

2. Look in a mirror. Let your eyes go out of focus. Look just past your head and shoulders. Do you see a sort of shimmering mist? This is part of your aura.

3. This exercise can be done with a group. Take turns standing in front of a blank wall. A white wall is probably the best choice here. The group looks at the individual standing in front of the wall. We may refer to that person as the subject. If you are taking the role of observer, allow your eyes to go softly out of focus, as above. Notice if you observe a shimmering glow or perhaps a light fog around the subject's head and shoulders. If you are the subject, there are two things you can do, one after the other:

Think of happy moments. Then think of sad or otherwise unpleasant moments. Observers: what do you notice happening to the subject's aura? Here's something else for the subject to do: visualize an object such as a bird or flower. Ask if anyone in the group can guess what you are thinking of or "outpicturing."

4. To sense energy: Rub your hands together fifteen to twenty times. Then pull them apart so the palms face each other with a distance of half an inch between them. What do you notice? Perhaps a sponginess? A light tingling or warmth? Someone has described the feeling as one of resistance. This is your energy. Slowly pull your hands apart. Gradually move them so they are still facing each other but each hand is about a foot from your waist. Notice if there are alternating layers of warmth and coolness. Very likely you are sensing layers of your aura.

5. Here is an exercise you can do with a partner. Take turns being a sender and a recipient. The sender sends unconditional love to the recipient. When you as the receiver receive unconditional love, hug the

sender. How you conceive of unconditional love is up to you. When I was introduced to this exercise, I quickly thought of a few possibilities and used them all before finding something that consistently worked well for me: visualizing myself as a ball of white light and sending white light to my respective partners.

6. Pay attention to colors. One possible exercise involves taking turns with a partner. The receiver in this case is blindfolded. The sender hands the receiver various swatches of cloth of different colors. The idea is for the receiver to describe impressions, whether in terms of feelings, images and the like. There is the option of guessing the color but the impressions are probably of greater interest and significance. Once the recipient has described impressions, the blindfold can be removed. Note: colors take on different meanings when not associated with auras. White itself is a combination of all colors. You might notice this when shining a light into a prism. In contrast, black is the absence of color. Some associate black with mystery, messages and whatever is hidden

or occult. The word occult itself means "hidden," not necessarily bad or evil. It is interesting to note how some people respond to black clothing or black walls. Speaking personally, I feel very drained when I am in a room with black walls and am all too glad to leave it as soon as possible. Then there are various colors. Blue may be associated with calm in one context and depression in another. And again, there are different shades and hues of red. One shade may suggest anger while another suggests passion, will and drive. Perhaps the best rule of thumb for this exercise is: suspend judgment. Allow impressions to flow, without attempting to interpret them.

Note: When I suggest allowing impressions to flow, I am referring to intuition. In order for you to access your intuition, you need to bypass the analytical, logical frame of mind, also known as the "Chattering monkey mind." One way of doing this is through progressive relaxation. To do this, sit comfortably and breathe deeply from the diaphragm. In other words, breathe from your belly rather than from your chest.

Breathing from your diaphragm allows for deeper breaths. Focus on the top of your head and relax the muscles there. Then focus on the muscles of your forehead and relax them as well. Continue with the muscles around your eyes and ears, then move on down to your neck, your shoulders, arms and hands, your chest, your abdomen, your pelvis, buttocks, hips, thighs, calves, lower legs, feet and toes. If you have a favorite mantra, word or phrase, you may repeat it silently to yourself. One example of a useful phrase is "I am." Another is "I am peace." You may also inhale and say one phrase to yourself and exhale and add another phrase. Inhale and say to yourself, "I am" and exhale, saying "at peace" or any combination of words and sounds you find comforting. With your mind quieted and calmed, you are ready to approach exercises such as the one previously described from a more receptive standpoint.

7. Here is another color exercise, this time without cloth swatches. Take turns once again. This time, the sender visualizes light

of different colors and imagines sending beams of this light to the recipient. Once again, the recipient describes his or her impressions. Note: red, yellow and orange are "warm" colors while blue, green and purple are "cool" colors. The recipient might comment on these differences if you send one example after the other.

8. There are probably a variety of exercises one can do with chakras. Some forms of Yoga involve visualizing the chakras, as well as energy flowing upward and past them. The energy is called Kundalini and is associated with enlightenment. The subjects of yoga and enlightenment are different from the content of this book. Let us consider one particular exercise though: how musical notes correspond to the chakras. One approach is to find a way to listen to various pitches and notice where in your body you feel the sound. Having a piano or keyboard handy might help. Then again, you can download sound samples from the internet. Another approach is to notice where you feel the sounds of various instruments. You might feel the sounds of drums, especially bass drums in your root

chakras while you feel the sounds of piccolo in your ears or even at the top of your head!

Working on yourself; some more information about Level 1

I will now describe the hand positions for Level 1 and include a short visualization/meditation.

The first hand position is at the top of the head. You may place your hands parallel to one another. Move them to the back of your head. This is the second position. Along with this arrangement, there is the option of covering your eyes and then your ears (or vice versa), even though doing so adds two other hand positions. That is okay too. You may be thorough here. At the same time, you might want to consider: energy goes to where it is needed. The third hand position is at the throat and neck. You might want to hold your hands at either side of your neck. Then place your hands at the center of your chest. Move them down to your solar plexus, near the bottom of your rib cage. The sacral chakra is located two inches below the navel. Place your hands there. Whether you move them further down to the lowest chakra is up to you. You might also want to place your hands on your knees and ankles. Even though the chakras in those joints are not among the seven major ones, I still occasionally direct Reiki energy there when I feel it is appropriate.

Give yourself the gift of self-healing

Where your attention and intention go, there your energy flows.

Give yourself ten to fifteen minutes for this meditation. Find a quiet place where you will not be disturbed. Put your cellphone on silent and eliminate other distractions if at all possible. Sit down in a comfortable chair. Close your eyes. Relax. Breathe deeply. Imagine a white ball of light above your head. Visualize it sending a beam of light into the top of your head and filling your body. Imagine roots growing from the

bottom of your feet and into the ground,
deep into Mother Earth. Imagine a gigantic
emerald green crystal in the center of the
Earth. Visualize green light traveling up the
roots and into the bottom of your feet and
then up to your heart.

Now visualize the white and green light
mixing. The white represents unconditional
love and the green represents healing.
Mentally direct the two colors to the first
chakra, at the base of the spine. Imagine
the first chakra as a ball of red light. Then
move up to the sacral chakra. Imagine that
as an orange ball of light. Continue to the
third chakra at the solar plexus. Imagine a
ball of yellow light. Move on up to the heart
center and visualize an emerald green ball
of light there. Then keep going to the throat
chakra, a lovely eggshell or sky blue color.
Continue to the middle of your forehead,
the third eye. Visualize a ball of indigo:
midnight blue. Then visualize a purple
flower with many petals at the top of your
head. Perhaps the lotus comes to mind.
This is an appropriate example. Now add a
layer of silver around your body. Silver

represents intuition, receptivity and the feminine aspect. It is also a protective color, being reflective. Add a layer of gold, for wisdom and the masculine aspect. Wrap yourself with a cocoon of white light for additional protection and add splashes of magenta and pink for unconditional love. Sit with these images for a few minutes and then slowly come back to the room. I will count backwards from ten to one and when I have reached one, you will be back, rested and refreshed. Take your time returning. 10, 9, 8, 7, 6. Wiggle your fingers and toes. 5,4. Coming back slowly. 3, 2, 1. Open your eyes. Welcome back. When you work with energy, especially with Reiki, you are likely to feel "spaced out" afterwards. That is, you may feel light headed. Perhaps also, you will feel like going to the restroom more often than usual. This is normal. Energy goes to where it is needed. Very likely, whatever blockages you had are being cleared. Probably the best thing to do is drink a lot of water. This is what I advise clients who request I do Reiki sessions with them.

My take on Level 2

With level 2, the student learns how to heal others. In my experience, I learned how to work with people but after reading a few books about Reiki with animals, I extended my practice to work with pets and an occasional wild animal when appropriate. The hand positions for working with people are similar to the ones you use for working on yourself. As for Reiki with animals, I feel that is a separate topic and will consider it further on.

When it comes to Level 2, ethics come to mind. There are a number of guidelines to consider. Not all Reiki practitioners are physicians (aka, doctors). Prescribing medications and treatments without a license to practice medicine is illegal. Also, it is not up to a Reiki practitioner to diagnose or treat a disease or condition. We can only do what we can to help a client (or patient, if you will) feel better. What we do is probably limited to laying on hands, sending healing energy and counseling, as appropriate.

Not everyone likes to be physically touched. Asking permission to touch someone is a good rule of thumb. At the same time, some parts of the body are off limits when it comes to physical contact: buttocks and private parts of both genders, as well as a woman's breasts. Do not place hands or fingers directly on a person's throat. Doing so resembles choking or strangling. Very likely you can do well by placing your hands lightly to either side of the neck or on the back of the neck.

Reiki energy is not limited by time, space or distance. Physical touch is not really needed. You can direct Reiki to where it needs to go even by holding your hands above the person's body. With this in mind, it is unwise to advise a client to disrobe. People who profess to practice Reiki and urge their clients to remove clothing are acting in a disreputable manner!

Also, there is good reason to ask permission before giving a healing session. Not everyone is ready to be healed. Some do not even want to be healed. There is such thing as free will and it needs to be respected. There is nothing wrong with sending love since we all need love. But when it comes to sending healing energy, doing so without a person's consent may have some unpleasant consequences.

Something else worth noting: Reiki hand positions are the same whether you work on a person's front or back. Except for the buttocks, touching the person's back is a lot less risky than touching anywhere on his or her front.

There are other ethical guidelines to consider, including practitioner/client confidentiality. Discussing clients' "issues" with other people is definitely unwise. This sort of talk is akin to gossip and may have serious consequences for the practitioner. Likewise claiming you can heal or cure something or otherwise boasting.

I have heard of cases where practitioners sent Reiki energy to a medical condition. The problem with this approach is it gives power to them, rather than to a person's health. This is similar to some physicians waging war on disease. Instead of conquering the disease they are merely perpetuating it. The goal of healing is to restore a person's sense of wholeness and wellbeing. Playing God is not part of the equation.

If there is one thing I have learned in my practice, it is humility. Here are the Reiki Principles, as I have learned them.

Just for today, do not anger.

Just for today, do not worry.

Just for today, earn your living honestly.

Just for today, show gratitude to every living thing.

Just for today, Honor your parents, teachers and elders.

The third principle might also read: Just for today, I do the best job I can.

Distant or absent healing

I have conducted healing sessions in person, as well as using the telephone and the internet. Sometimes I have done what I felt was appropriate and contacted my client afterwards for feedback. Sometimes I imagine the client is in front of me and place my hands in the air as if I was conducting a one to one healing sessions. Other times I will imagine myself as a white ball of light and mentally direct healing energy to my client. I have heard of cases where one can use a substitute such as a doll and mentally direct healing energy to a person using the doll as a focal point. Once again, intention plays a major part in the process: 99 percent intention and one percent technique.

About technique, or rather techniques. I am in the habit of drawing Reiki symbols over the heads of clients when I am finishing a session. I also make cutting motions in the air and snap my fingers. I learned these little rituals from observing my teachers and other practitioners. One of my teachers also claps her hands and blows puffs of air around her clients. Sometimes she also grabs at what seem like empty air and either pulls or pushes the handfuls away. Snapping fingers and clapping hands are ways of breaking up stagnant energy, even if only on a symbolic level. What seems like grabbing empty air and making cutting motions are removing symbolic blocks and attachments. Blowing air may represent making positive, supportive ideas the client's own or getting stagnant energy moving again. All these rituals may seem bizarre to an observer but if they work for the practitioner, that is fine, too. Reiki is an intuitive art. Once again, intention is the most important factor to consider. What works for one practitioner may not work for another practitioner.

Reiki and animals

Cats and dogs seem to take well to Reiki. There are a few guidelines to keep in mind. Ask a pet's permission before conducting a session. Yes, that is what I wrote. Ask permission. Animals are not stupid, contrary to what some people seem to think. Also, you might want to conduct distance healing sessions to begin with. Not every pet likes to be touched or handled and this goes for any pet, especially if he or she is not yours. The same goes for wild animals as well as pets. Furthermore, there is a distinction between cats and dogs. Cats don't seem to appreciate having their abdomens touched, even if dogs enjoy a good belly rub. You might do well with touching a pet's head, chest or back. In general, pets seem to have a way of telling you if they want Reiki. They could back into your hands or rub against them. A session may end not when you think it is over but when the pet signals to you it is so by simply walking away or licking your hands ("kissing" in the manner of pets). I sometimes imagine my heart as a green emerald and when I meet someone else's pet, I visualize a similar gem at the animal's heart center, along with a beam of light connecting the two jewels. This is a symbolic way of establishing a "heart to heart" connection and forming a sort of emotional bond. Whether I send healing or not, at least I have made a new friend and/or maintained the friendship.

Sometimes a pet can show appreciation in an interesting way. One of my shoulders sometimes aches. I recently discovered one possible reason is osteoarthritis. Once I had a kitten and the little fellow climbed onto my affected shoulder and lay there for quite a while, purring loudly. His body heat had an effect similar to that of a heating pad. The continuous sound of his purring was comforting as well.

Reiki with plants, the Earth and situations

I have heard of Reiki being used to encourage plant growth, to heal the Earth and to promote beneficial outcomes of various situations. Personally, I have used Reiki with plants in and around my house. How effective is what I do? I don't know but I do it anyway. You might want to consider an experiment where you have two groups of plants, one as a control and the other as an experimental group. Send Reiki to the experimental group and give no treatment to the control group. Just water and otherwise care for each group as you would any other plants and see which group sprouts faster and/or grows faster. As for how effective other uses for Reiki are, I am not sure but figure if it contributes to the wellbeing of all it is worth doing.

The Master level

With Level three, one has the option of teaching Reiki to others. Then again, being a Reiki master suggests one is the master of one's own life. Self-mastery is an ongoing process. Sometimes that is mastery enough. Teaching can be challenging. The best I could do is probably show a person he is his own best teacher. What you learn as a student is what you learn. I doubt I can teach you anything. I can only show you my way and what works for me. What works for me may not work for some people. One of my teacher often says, "We are all works in progress." That makes sense to me.

Healing on the physical, mental, emotional and spiritual levels

The way I think of myself as a healer is, I am a channel of healing energy. I merely step out of the way. A physician can only dress the wound. The body heals itself. This is true, even though I dress no physical wounds and I am not a physician. Healing work gives the sender and the receiver both a feeling of wellbeing. It is as much a healing for the sender as it is for the receiver. Along with the physical, there may be healing at the mental and emotional levels. A simpler way of describing this is the healing of beliefs, also known as thoughts with expectations attached. Part of what I do involves intuitive counseling. When one changes the way he or she thinks, one changes his or her experiences, as well as his or her own reality.

A guided meditation/visualization I have often used with students

Imagine sitting in a circle with other people. Visualize yourself as a being of light. Imagine all people around the circle as beings of light as well. Now imagine there is an emerald green jewel at your heart center. Visualize green light going around the circle, connecting everyone's heart center in a large ring. Now send another beam of light into the center of the circle. Imagine where the beams cross there is another ball of light that grows larger and larger until the entire space is contained within that ball of light. Now that ball of light expands until it contains your city, then your state, then the entire country and then the entire world. If you wish you can extend that ball of light until it contains the solar system, the galaxy and even the universe or universes if you will conceive of many universes. That green light is healing energy. Imagine it touch every sentient being and healing them. Imagine that light filling your body and healing you, rejuvenating you, down to the cellular level.

Now if you wish, say aloud or think about any sentient being, whether human or otherwise, that comes to mind who may benefit from healing, with the understanding it is up to him or her to accept that healing. Also hold the intention this healing energy be used for the highest good of all.

Be sure to keep some healing energy for yourself. We are only effective as healers as we ourselves our healthy. Sit with the images as you wish.

Continue to send healing energy to those who need it. I now include Gaia, also known as Pachamama and Mother Earth herself, on the list.

I will now call us back, counting from ten to one. Be sure to ground yourself. Adding the image of yourself as a tree, with roots growing into the ground and branches reaching into the sky, may help. 10, 9, 8, 7, 6, 5, 4, 3, 2, 1. Open your eyes.

Welcome back.

The use of tools

Some Reiki practitioners use tools such as aromatic oils and or crystals as part of their work. I rarely tools myself. Most of the time I use my hands and mind. I do have a collection of quartz crystals and other semi-precious stones in my house, though. Sometimes I will pick up a selenite or quartz crystal wand for the purpose of sending healing energy to someone who needs it. Otherwise, my collection seems to enhance the peaceful atmosphere of the house. In that regard, they serve their purpose.

More exercises:

1. This is a variation of the sensing energy exercise. Rub your hands together fifteen to twenty times. Gently pull your hands apart so there is a gap of about half an inch between them. Be sure to breathe deeply while you do this. Inhale through your nose and exhale through your mouth. Now imagine there is a little ball of light between the palms of your hands. Pull your hands apart an inch further and visualize the ball become larger. Now slowly continue pulling your hands apart and imagine the ball increases to the size of a baseball or even the size of a basketball. How large you make the ball depends on your preferences, as well as how far apart you can comfortably pull your hands. Now play catch with yourself, visualizing the ball bouncing between the palms. Notice if you feel the ball striking each hand. The sensation, if any, is subtle but very likely it is there! Have fun doing this. It is high play. Now think about unconditional love and what it means to you. Imagine what it is like to be unconditionally loved. Put that into the ball. Send unconditional love into the ball by imagining the feeling going there. Images, feelings, smells, sounds, tastes or any combination of

those senses may come to mind. Someone told me her conception of unconditional love tasted, looked and smelled like cotton candy. That is perfectly fine. Now, having sent a good sized dose of unconditional love into the ball, grasp it with both hands and bring it to your heart center. Press the ball to yourself and imagine it melting into your very being. Really breathe deeply. Notice what it is like to give yourself the gift of unconditional love, that is, to love yourself. This too, is an important part of healing.

2. Repeat exercise 1. This time, send the ball of light to anyone who comes to mind. Asking permission before sending healing energy is a good rule of thumb but there certainly is no such restriction when it comes to sending unconditional love.

3. Send light and love to the beverages you drink and foods you eat. Notice how much better you feel after doing this. I say "thank you" every time I eat a meal or drink a glass of water. Part of my Reiki practice includes generous doses of gratitude.

4. Someone guided me this exercise as a sort of mini-workshop. She advised me to use a particular stone called a Chrysocolla. When I

followed through, I felt a slight headache for just a minute or thereabouts but the sensation passed quickly. You may use a Chrysocolla (a light green stone), a clear quartz crystal or a selenite wand. Please do this exercise standing. Close your eyes. Breathe deeply. Inhale through your nose and exhale through your mouth. Hold the crystal with your right hand. I suggest the right hand because to me, the right side of the body is the active and "sending" side while the left is the receptive and "receiving" side. Point the crystal toward the base of your spine, near the tail bone. Keep the crystal there for about half a minute, then move it up so it is two inches below your navel. Continue raising your hand so the crystal is pointing at your solar plexus, then your heart center, your throat and middle of your forehead. Keep breathing. When your hand reaches overhead, instead of continuing to point the crystal, wave both hands in an up and down circular motion. You might notice sensations of congestion in various parts of your body during this process, including mild sinus congestion and a slight headache. In my experience, these feelings pass quickly. What you have done is a sort of self-healing exercise, using the crystal. One way to enhance the experience is to repeat this procedure, visualizing white light passing through the crystal and clearing any blockages in your chakras.

5. This exercise may work with colored semi-precious stones or colored stones. It is based on the concept of "laying on of stones." Collect seven stones. They may be small rocks or pebbles you find by a stream, stones you buy at a local metaphysical bookstore or anything of that nature, as long as they are clean and you feel comfortable with them. Find time when you will be alone and undisturbed. Lie down on a bed, couch, the floor or wherever you can be comfortable. Place the stones in the following arrangement: red on or close to your tail bone, orange two inches below your navel, yellow on your solar plexus, green at the center of your chest, blue at your throat, indigo on your forehead and purple just over your head. Relax and breathe. Visualize your chakras: the root, sacral, solar plexus, heart center, throat, third eye and crown, all as colored balls of light. Add bubbles of white, silver and gold light for protection, along with magenta and pink for unconditional love. Imagine the stones are

absorbing all the stresses and strains of the day and helping you release the effect of painful memories and other forms of "negativity." Imagine the stones helping you achieve a sense of balance and peace. When you are ready, come back to the room. Remove the stones. You may want to wash them to symbolically remove any negativity associated with them.

The Healing state of mind

Part of healing refers to a state of mind. One may be or seem healthy physically but not so healthy mentally or emotionally. Holding onto anger and similar emotions is not particularly healthy. Then again, neither are obsessions: thinking the same thoughts over and over again, repeatedly. One definition of emotion I have heard is "energy in motion." As for anger, there is nothing wrong with it in and of itself, as long as it is expressed in a constructive way. Anger at injustice is understandable. As for other emotions, there is nothing inherently good or bad about them either. When I have done healing work, some clients cry or laugh. Crying and laughing are emotional releases, as far as I am concerned. Unfortunately, some of us have been taught not to cry or laugh. Or perhaps we have been discouraged from laughing loudly. To me, this "repression" in the name of social approval is unhealthy and destructive. One aspect of healing is to address questionable assumptions and let them go.

When I talk about mental healing I talk about healing of beliefs. One definition of belief is "a thought with expectations attached. When you change your beliefs, you change the nature of your experiences. One exercise is to keep a journal of your beliefs. This way, you can keep track of whatever may be holding you back and otherwise limiting you. You can change a belief by substituting its opposite. What I am talking about are affirmations. These are positive, uplifting words and phrases stated in the present tense.

Reiki as natural healing

To me, good health relates to being at peace, in harmony and "in the flow." It is a state of mind. As we think, so we are. This seems to be in contrast with the Western medicine concept of health being the absence of disease or a battle against disease. Health cannot be measured or reduced down to numbers. My experiences with Reiki have included references to Nature, natural settings and natural objects. Going for walks when the weather is pleasant is healing in and of itself. I sometimes advise my clients to imagine waterfalls. Such images are tranquilizers in and of themselves. The images are free and there are no side effects!

Releasing exercises

1. This is a variation of a meditation/visualization I learned from one of my teachers. A few years ago, I attended a conference where the presenter described the Ancient Egyptian Fire Ceremony. In the Ceremony, initiates walk through a fire but are not burned. Only their weaknesses are consumed. Perhaps the ceremony is symbolic, rather than literal. The ceremony seems to be very much like the meditation I am about to describe. I do not know whether my teacher is familiar with the ceremony itself, by the way.

Find a place where you will not be disturbed
for the next ten to fifteen minutes. If you have
a cellphone, put it on silent or Airplane mode.
Sit in a comfortable chair and close your eyes.
Relax. Breathe deeply. Inhale through your
nose and exhale through your mouth.

Imagine sitting on a rocky plateau. The sun is
shining and there is a warm breeze. You are
safe here. Directly in front of you there is a
wood bowl. Also in front of you and a few feet
away there is a fire. To either side there are
piles of stones. I am going to read you a list of
words. Some of these words may push buttons,
in a sense. That is, they will remind you of
unpleasant situations and memories. If any of
these words trigger off something in you, pick
up a stone and put it in the bowl. If you notice
no reaction to a word, let it go. "If it does not
apply, let it fly," as my teacher often says.
Abortion: aborted child; aborted plans.
Addictions. Addictions to drugs, habits,
relationships, etc. Anger. Anxiety. Bullying,
Bullies. Carelessness. Deceit and deception.
Denial. Despair. Discrimination.
Disappointment. Fear you have been
discriminated against. Depression. Fear.

Frustration. Greed. Guilt. Hate. Helplessness. Hopelessness. Hostility. Judgment. Loss. Malice. Manipulation. Neediness. Rejection. Revenge. Sarcasm. Shame. Victimhood. Feeling you are a victim.

Other words and associated memories and the feelings associated with the memories may surface. If so, place stones in the bowl as appropriate.
Now take a look at the bowl and its contents. Are they piled high? Do you see a pile of sand, gravel, small stones or even boulders? I leave plenty of leeway in terms of interpretation of how large to make the bowl and stones!

While looking at the bowl here is the next step. Say aloud or to yourself:
"I see you. I recognize you and accept you but I am not you. Perhaps I can say I am grateful for having you in my life because if it wasn't for you, I would not be the person I am today. I no longer need you. I am not my thoughts, my feelings, or my body. I am (state your name) and I am present." Now see yourself lifting that bowl and hurling it and its contents into the

fire. Observe the bowl and stones burning up and vanishing.

Nature abhors a vacuum. Imagine any spaces left from releasing all those burdens glowing with white light. You may extend the visual image to seeing your entire body glowing with this light.

Here are a couple of affirmations you might want to consider repeating to yourself: "I am light. I am love." The statements may seem corny but repeat them a few times and notice how and what you feel.

2. For this exercise, you will visualize a pool. The image of a swimming pool is fine if you prefer. Imagine walking through the woods on a sunny day. The birds are singing and there is a gentle breeze. As you continue walking, you notice a clearing. Go to that clearing. There you will find a pool. This is your pool. Nobody else is about. Here you may take off your clothes or change into a bathing suit, if you prefer. Perhaps the pool has steps, a ladder or both. For ease of description, let us consider steps. Imagine sticking your foot into the pool at the

shallow end. Notice how warm or cool the water is. If you like, you can imagine the water is warm. Step further into the pool. Wade or swim, as you wish. Take your time. After a while, you may wish to lie on your back and let the water support your weight. Allow it to buoy you up. Gaze in the sky and passing clouds, if you like. Imagine the tensions of the day as sand, being washed away and floating to the bottom of the pool, to be transformed into light. Consider how much the human body is made up of water and how it feels to be one with water. Feel what it is like to be connected to other people and other beings. When you are ready, stand up and make your way to the shallow end of the pool again. Step out. Close by, there is a towel for you. Dry yourself off and put your clothes back on. Find your way to the path and walk through the woods, to the place where you started. When you are ready, come back to the room and open your eyes.

Namaste.

www.ingramcontent.com/pod-product-compliance
Lightning Source LLC
Chambersburg PA
CBHW070237290526

45789CB00004B/1657